LOW-CARB DIET PLAN COOK BOOK

A Comprehensive Manual on the Low-Carb Diet: Boost Your Energy Levels through the Low-Carb Diet

REX LEWIS

Table of Contents

Introduction

Low-Carb Diets Limit Carbohydrate Intake While Focusing On Larger Amounts of Proteins and Lipids. Low-Carb Diets Aim To Promote The Body's Utilization Of Stored Fat For Energy, Resulting In Weight Loss. Various Types Of Low-Carb Diets Include The Ketogenic Diet, Atkins Diet, And Low-Carbohydrate, High-Fat (LCHF) Diet.

Below Are Fundamental Principles And Components Of Low-Carb Diets:

• Carbohydrate Restriction Is The Primary Feature Of Low-Carb Diets, Involving A Decrease In Carbohydrate Consumption. Carbohydrates Are Present In Foods Such As Grains, Starchy Vegetables, Fruits, And

Legumes. These Diets Usually Focus On Foods High In Protein And Beneficial Fats.

• Ketosis Is Targeted By Certain Low-Carb Diets, Such As The Ketogenic Diet. Ketosis Is The Metabolic State In Which The Body Depletes Its Glycogen Stores And Begins Converting Lipids Into Ketones As An Alternative Source Of Energy. This Process Can Lead To Weight Reduction, Enhanced Mental Acuity, And Regulated Blood Glucose Levels.

• Protein Is An Essential Element In Low-Carb Diets. It Aids In Feeling Full, Maintains Muscular Mass, And Is Involved In Other Biological Functions. Primary Protein Sources In Low-Carb

Diets Are Meat, Poultry, Fish, Eggs, And Dairy Products.

• Low-Carb Diets Promote The Intake Of Good Fats Such As Avocados, Nuts, Seeds, Olive Oil, And Fatty Fish, Unlike Conventional Low-Fat Diets. Dietary Fat Contributes To Satiety And Can Act As A Main Fuel For The Body.

• Fiber Is Emphasized In Many Low-Carb Diets Due To Its Presence In Non-Starchy Vegetables, Despite The Restriction On Carbohydrates. Fiber Is Crucial For Digestive Health And Helps Mitigate Some Digestive Problems That May Result From A Low-Carb Diet.

- **Potential Health Benefits:** Low-Carb Diets Are Linked To Health Advantages Such As Weight Loss, Enhanced Blood Sugar Regulation, And Improved Lipid Profiles. Low-Carb Diets Are Beneficial For Those With Diseases Such As Metabolic Syndrome And Type 2 Diabetes.

- **Individual Variability:** It Is Crucial To Recognize That Reactions To Low-Carb Diets Might Differ Among Individuals. Some Individuals Excel On These Diets, Achieving Weight Loss And Enhanced Health Indicators, While Others May Not React Well To Them.

Low-Carb Diets Are Successful For Short-Term Weight Loss But Can Be

Tough For Certain Persons To Maintain In The Long Term. It Is Essential To Discover A Nutritional Regimen That Is Sustainable For Each Individual's Lifestyle And Tastes.

Prior To Making Substantial Dietary Adjustments, It Is Recommended To Get Guidance From A Healthcare Expert Or A Qualified Dietitian To Confirm That The Selected Method Is In Line With Your Health Requirements And Objectives. It Is Crucial To Check Nutritional Intake And Maintain Hydration While Following Any Diet Plan.

CHAPTER ONE
Who Can Benefit From A Low-Carb Diet?

The Effectiveness Of A Low-Carb Diet Might Vary Based On An Individual's Health Objectives, Medical Issues, And Personal Choices. Here Are Several Demographics That May Benefit From A Low-Carb Diet:

- **Individuals Seeking Weight Loss:** Low-Carbohydrate Diets Are Frequently Successful For Reducing Weight. Decreasing Carbohydrate Consumption Prompts The Body To Utilize Stored Fat For Energy, Resulting In Weight Loss. Higher Consumption Of Protein And Fat Can Lead To A Sensation Of Satiety, Which

In Turn Decreases The Total Number Of Calories Consumed.

• Low-Carb Diets Are Good For Persons With Type 2 Diabetes Since They Can Help Manage Blood Sugar Levels Effectively. Restricting Carbohydrates Reduces The Need For Insulin And Can Lead To More Stable Blood Sugar Levels.

• Individuals With Metabolic Syndrome Or Insulin Resistance May Find A Low-Carb Diet Beneficial. These Diseases Are Typically Marked By Increased Blood Sugar Levels, Raised Blood Pressure, And Aberrant Lipid Profiles, Which Can Be Alleviated By Reducing Carbohydrate Intake.

• Women With Polycystic Ovary Syndrome (Pcos), A Hormonal Condition, May Benefit From A Low-Carb Diet To Help Control Symptoms Like Insulin Resistance, Weight Gain, And Irregular Menstrual Cycles.

• The Ketogenic Diet, Which Is Very Low In Carbohydrates And High In Fats, Is Utilized As A Therapeutic Method For Treating Epilepsy, Especially In Children. It Can Potentially Decrease The Occurrence And Intensity Of Seizures.

• Some People With Specific Cardiovascular Risk Concerns, Such Elevated Triglycerides And Reduced Hdl Cholesterol Levels, Can Find A Low-Carb Diet Advantageous. It Is

Essential To Prioritize Selecting Healthy Fats And Keeping Track Of Overall Nutritional Consumption.

• Endurance Athletes May Choose For Low-Carb Or Ketogenic Diets For Training In A Low-Glycogen Condition, Despite The Normal Need For Carbohydrates For Energy Among Athletes. Nevertheless, Individual Reactions Can Differ, And These Diets May Not Be Appropriate For All Individuals.

• The Ketogenic Diet Has Been Studied For Its Possible Cognitive Advantages And Neuroprotective Properties Related To Brain Health. Some Studies Indicate Potential Therapeutic Use For

Neurodegenerative Illnesses, But Further Research Is Required.

Individual Reactions To A Low-Carb Diet Can Vary, And Benefits May Not Be Uniform For Everyone. Prior To Making Substantial Dietary Adjustments, It Is Advisable For Individuals To Seek Guidance From Healthcare Professionals Or Trained Dietitians, Particularly If They Have Current Medical Illnesses Or Concerns. Long-Term Commitment To A Diet Is Important For Lasting Results, Therefore It's Critical To Select A Method That Matches Personal Preferences And Lifestyle.

Advantages of a Low-Carb Lifestyle

Embracing A Low-Carbohydrate Lifestyle Can Provide Numerous Health Advantages For Specific Individuals. Here Are Some Potential Benefits Of Adhering To A Low-Carbohydrate Diet:

• Weight Loss Is A Primary Motivation For Individuals Adopting A Low-Carb Lifestyle. Decreasing Carbohydrate Consumption Causes The Body To Transition To Utilizing Stored Fat For Energy, Resulting In Weight Reduction.

• Low-Carb Diets Can Enhance Blood Sugar Regulation, Which Is Especially Advantageous For Those With Insulin

Resistance, Prediabetes, Or Type 2 Diabetes. Restricting Carbohydrate Consumption Reduces The Need For Insulin And Can Help Regulate Blood Sugar Levels.

• Adopting A Low-Carb Diet Can Decrease The Likelihood Of Getting Type 2 Diabetes, Particularly For Individuals With Predisposed Factors Like Obesity Or A Family History Of The Condition.

• Some Research Indicates That Low-Carb Diets Can Enhance Heart Health By Improving Cardiovascular Risk Factors, Including Lowering Triglycerides, Raising Hdl (Good) Cholesterol Levels, And Enhancing Overall Lipid Profiles. The Kind And

Quality Of Fats Consumed Significantly Impact Cardiovascular Health.

• Protein And Fat-Rich Foods In A Low-Carb Diet Can Increase Feelings Of Fullness And Decrease Total Calorie Consumption, Thereby Improving Appetite Control.

• Enhanced Cognitive Function: Some People Experience Increased Mental Focus And Clarity While Adhering To A Low-Carb Or Ketogenic Diet. Ketosis Can Generate Ketones That Serve As An Alternate Fuel For The Brain.

• Some Low-Carb Diets, Especially Those Focusing On Full, Unprocessed Foods, Can Reduce Inflammation. Chronic Inflammation Is Associated

With Range Of Health Problems, Such As Metabolic Syndrome And Cardiovascular Disease.

• Low-Carb Diets Typically Result In Improved Triglyceride Levels, Which Is Advantageous For Heart Health. High Levels Of Triglycerides Are Linked To A Higher Likelihood Of Developing Cardiovascular Illnesses.

• Management Of Pcos Symptoms: Women With Polycystic Ovarian Syndrome (Pcos) May See Betterment In Symptoms Including Irregular Menstrual Periods And Insulin Resistance By Adopting A Low-Carb Lifestyle.

• The Ketogenic Diet, Characterized By Very Low Carbohydrate And High Fat Intake, Has Shown Promise For Therapeutic Use In Medical Disorders Such As Epilepsy, Neurological Diseases, And Some Types Of Cancer.

It's Crucial To Recognize That Although A Low-Carb Lifestyle Can Provide These Advantages For Certain Persons, It May Not Be Appropriate For Everyone. Emphasizing Full, Nutrient-Dense Foods Is Essential For General Health Since The Quality Of Food Choices Plays A Significant Role. Prior To Making Substantial Dietary Alterations, It Is Advisable For Individuals To Seek Guidance From Healthcare Professionals Or Trained

Dietitians, Particularly If They Have Current Medical Illnesses Or Concerns.

Stocking Your Low-Carb Kitchen

Stocking Your Kitchen With The Right Foods Is Crucial For Successfully Maintaining A Low-Carb Lifestyle. Here's A List Of Foods That Are Typically Suitable For A Low-Carb Diet:

Proteins:

- Chicken, Turkey, Beef, Pork, Lamb, And Other Meats
- Fish And Seafood
- Eggs
- Tofu And Tempeh (For Vegetarians)

Healthy Fats:

- Olive Oil

- Avocado Oil

- Coconut Oil

- Butter And Ghee

- Nuts And Seeds (Almonds, Walnuts, Chia Seeds, Flaxseeds)

Low-Carb Vegetables:

- Leafy Greens (Spinach, Kale, Lettuce, Arugula)

- Cruciferous Vegetables (Broccoli, Cauliflower, Brussels Sprouts)

- Zucchini

- Bell Peppers

- Asparagus

Low-Sugar Fruits:

- Berries (Strawberries, Blueberries, Raspberries)
- Avocados
- Lemons And Limes

Dairy:

- Cheese (Cheddar, Mozzarella, Feta, Cream Cheese)
- Greek Yogurt (Unsweetened)
- Heavy Cream
- Butter

Nuts and Seeds:

- Almonds
- Walnuts
- Chia Seeds
- Flaxseeds

- Pumpkin Seeds

Low-Carb Sweeteners:

- Stevia

- Erythritol

- Monk Fruit

Condiments And Sauces:

- Mustard

- Mayonnaise (Check For Added Sugars)

- Vinegar (Balsamic, Apple Cider)

- Soy Sauce Or Tamari (For A Gluten-Free Option)

- Hot Sauce

Herbs And Spices:

- Basil

- Oregano

- Cumin

- Paprika

- Garlic Powder

Other Pantry Staples:

- Coconut Flour And Almond Flour (For Low-Carb Baking)

- Unsweetened Almond Milk Or Coconut Milk

- Canned Tuna Or Salmon

- Broth Or Stock (Check For Added Sugars)

- Dark Chocolate With A High Cocoa Content (In Moderation)

When Setting Up Your Low-Carb Kitchen, It Is Crucial To Meticulously Scrutinize Labels, Since Certain Items Could Include Concealed Sugars Or

Undesirable Ingredients. Moreover, Prioritize Consuming Complete, Unprocessed Foods To Provide A Diverse Intake Of Nutrients.

Consider That Individual Tolerance To Carbohydrates Can Differ, So Tailor Your Options According To Your Personal Dietary Requirements And Objectives. For Tailored Advise About Specific Health Concerns Or Medical Conditions, It Is Recommended To Consult With A Healthcare Expert Or A Qualified Dietitian.

CHAPTER TWO
What Are Carbohydrates?

Carbohydrates Are A Primary Macronutrient, Along With Proteins And Fats, That Supply Energy For The Body. Carbohydrates Are Organic Substances Composed Of Carbon, Hydrogen, And Oxygen Atoms. They Are Categorized Into Simple Carbohydrates (Sugars) And Complex Carbs (Starches And Fibers).

Simple Carbohydrates:

• **Monosaccharides:** These Are The Simplest Form Of Carbohydrates And Include Glucose, Fructose, And Galactose. These Single Sugar Molecules Are Quickly Absorbed By

The Body And Provide A Rapid Source Of Energy.

- **Disaccharides:** Disaccharides Are Composed Of Two Monosaccharide Units. Examples Include Sucrose (Glucose + Fructose), Lactose (Glucose + Galactose), and Maltose (Glucose + Glucose).

Complex Carbohydrates:

- **Polysaccharides:** These Are Large Molecules Made Up Of Multiple Monosaccharide Units. The Two Primary Types Are Starch And Glycogen.

- **Starch:** Found In Plants, Starch Is A Storage Form Of Energy. Common

Sources Include Grains, Legumes, And Tubers.

- **Glycogen:** This Is The Storage Form Of Glucose In Animals, Particularly In The Liver And Muscles.

- **Dietary Fiber:** Fiber Is A Type Of Complex Carbohydrate That The Body Cannot Fully Digest. It Is Classified Into Two Main Types:

- **Soluble Fiber:** Dissolves In Water And Can Help Lower Cholesterol Levels. Found In Fruits, Vegetables, And Legumes.

- **Insoluble Fiber:** Does Not Dissolve In Water And Adds Bulk To The Stool, Aiding In Digestion. Found In Whole Grains, Nuts, And Vegetables.

Carbohydrates Are Essential For The Body's Energy Metabolism. Upon Consumption, They Are Metabolized Into Glucose Or Other Monosaccharides, Which Cells Utilize As Their Main Energy Source. The Brain Is Highly Dependent On Glucose As Its Primary Source Of Energy.

Not All Carbohydrates Are Of The Same Quality, And The Source Of Carbohydrates Is Significant. Fruits, Vegetables, Whole Grains, And Legumes Are Nutritious Sources Of Carbs. Refined And Processed Carbs, Such Sweet Snacks And White Flour Products, May Lack Essential Nutrients And Lead To Health Problems If Taken Excessively. It Is

Recommended To Select Carbs That Are In Line With Your General Health And Lifestyle, As Individual Dietary Requirements And Objectives Can Differ.

Types of Carbohydrates

Carbohydrates Can Be Categorized Into Different Categories According To Their Chemical Composition And Metabolic Pathways In The Body. The Main Categories Consist Of Simple Carbohydrates (Sugars), Complex Carbohydrates (Starches And Fibers), And Sugar Alcohols. Here Is A Summary Of Each:

Simple Carbohydrates:

1. **Monosaccharides:** These Are Single Sugar Molecules.

2. **Glucose:** Often Referred To As Blood Sugar, It Is A Primary Source Of Energy For Cells.

3. **Fructose:** Found In Fruits And Honey.

4. **Galactose:** Found In Dairy Products.

5. **Disaccharides:** These Are Composed Of Two Monosaccharide Units.

6. **Sucrose:** Composed Of Glucose And Fructose; Found In Table Sugar.

7. **Lactose:** Composed Of Glucose And Galactose; Found In Milk.

8. **Maltose:** Composed Of Two Glucose Units; Found In Malted Foods.

Complex Carbohydrates:

1. **Polysaccharides:** These Are Larger Molecules Made Up Of Multiple Monosaccharide Units.
2. **Starch:** A Storage Form Of Energy In Plants, Found In Grains, Legumes, And Tubers.
3. **Glycogen:** A Storage Form Of Energy In Animals, Primarily Stored In The Liver And Muscles.

Dietary Fiber:

1. **Soluble Fiber:** Dissolves In Water And Can Help Lower

Cholesterol Levels. Found In Fruits, Vegetables, And Legumes.

2. **Insoluble Fiber:** Does Not Dissolve In Water And Adds Bulk To The Stool, Aiding In Digestion. Found In Whole Grains, Nuts, And Vegetables.

- **Sugar Alcohols (Polyols):** These Are Sugar Substitutes That Are Commonly Found In Sugar-Free And "Diet" Products. Examples Include Sorbitol, Xylitol, And Erythritol. Sugar Alcohols Have A Sweet Taste But Are Not Fully Absorbed By The Body, Resulting In Fewer Calories And Less Impact On Blood Sugar Levels.

• **Added Sugars:** These Are Sugars And Syrups That Are Added To Foods During Processing Or Preparation. Common Examples Include High-Fructose Corn Syrup, Sucrose, And Agave Nectar. Excessive Consumption Of Added Sugars Has Been Linked To Various Health Issues.

Understanding Various Carbohydrate Kinds Is Crucial. Opt For Full, Unadulterated Foods Over Refined And Sugary Options. Opting For Complex Carbs Like Whole Grains, Fruits, And Vegetables Offers Vital Nutrients And A Gradual Energy Release, Which Enhances General Health And Wellness. Individuals With Particular Health Concerns Or Dietary

Objectives Should Seek Advice From
Healthcare Professionals Or Qualified
Dietitians For Tailored
Recommendations.

CHAPTER THREE
Understanding the Workings of Low-Carb Diets

Low-Carb Diets Function By Greatly Decreasing Carbohydrate Consumption, Causing The Body To Switch Its Main Energy Source From Glucose (Obtained From Carbohydrates) To Stored Fat. Low-Carb Diets Mostly Work Through Certain Mechanisms Such As:

• **Inducing Ketosis:** Many Low-Carb Diets, Such As The Ketogenic Diet, Aim To Induce A State Of Ketosis. Ketosis Occurs When Carbohydrate Intake Is Restricted To The Point That The Body Begins To Rely On Fat For Fuel. In The Absence Of Sufficient Carbohydrates,

The Liver Converts Fats Into Ketones, Which Are Then Used As An Alternative Energy Source.

• **Reducing Insulin Levels:** Carbohydrate Consumption Leads To An Increase In Blood Sugar Levels, Triggering The Release Of Insulin, A Hormone That Helps Cells Take Up Glucose For Energy. Low-Carb Diets, By Restricting Carbohydrate Intake, Result In Lower Blood Sugar Levels, Reducing The Need For Insulin. This Can Be Particularly Beneficial For Individuals With Insulin Resistance Or Type 2 Diabetes.

- **Enhancing Fat Burning:** With Reduced Carbohydrate Availability, The Body Relies More On Stored Fat For Energy. This Can Lead To Increased Fat Burning, Resulting In Weight Loss. The Metabolic Shift Encourages The Breakdown Of Triglycerides (Stored Fat) Into Fatty Acids And Glycerol For Energy.

- **Appetite Regulation:** Low-Carb Diets Often Include Higher Amounts Of Protein And Fat, Which Can Contribute To Increased Feelings Of Fullness And Satiety. This May Lead To A Reduction In Overall Calorie Intake, Promoting Weight Loss.

• **Stabilizing Blood Sugar Levels:** By Minimizing The Consumption Of Rapidly Digestible Carbohydrates, Low-Carb Diets Can Help Stabilize Blood Sugar Levels. This Is Particularly Important For Individuals With Conditions Like Insulin Resistance Or Type 2 Diabetes.

• **Reducing Water Weight:** Glycogen, The Stored Form Of Glucose In The Muscles And Liver, Binds To Water. When Carbohydrate Intake Is Reduced, Glycogen Stores Are Depleted, Leading To A Loss Of Water Weight. While This Initial Weight Loss Is Often Rapid, It Primarily Involves Water Rather Than Fat.

The Efficacy Of Low-Carb Diets Can Differ Between Individuals Due To Factors Like Total Calorie Consumption, Food Content, And Individual Metabolic Reactions. Long-Term Commitment To A Low-Carbohydrate Lifestyle Is Essential For Maintaining Lasting Advantages.

Prior To Making Substantial Dietary Adjustments, It Is Advisable For Individuals To Seek Guidance From Healthcare Professionals Or Trained Dietitians, Particularly If They Have Current Medical Illnesses Or Concerns. It Is Crucial For Overall Health To Monitor Nutrient Consumption And Uphold A Balanced Diet.

Building Balanced Low-Carb Meals

To Create Well-Rounded Low-Carb Meals, Include Protein, Healthy Fats, And Non-Starchy Veggies While Limiting High-Carb Foods. Here Is A Comprehensive Guide To Assist You In Preparing Balanced And Fulfilling Low-Carbohydrate Meals:

Choose Protein Sources:

Include A Source Of Lean Protein In Each Meal. Options Include:

- Poultry (Chicken, Turkey)
- Lean Cuts Of Beef, Pork, Or Lamb
- Fish And Seafood
- Eggs

- Tofu Or Tempeh (For Vegetarians)
- Dairy Products (Cheese, Greek Yogurt)

Incorporate Healthy Fats:

Include Sources Of Healthy Fats To Add Flavor And Satiety. Examples Include:

- Avocado Or Guacamole
- Olive Oil
- Coconut Oil
- Nuts And Seeds (Almonds, Walnuts, Chia Seeds)
- Fatty Fish (Salmon, Mackerel)
- Butter Or Ghee

Choose Non-Starchy Vegetables:

Non-Starchy Vegetables Are Low In Carbohydrates And High In Fiber And Nutrients.

They Add Bulk To Your Meals Without Significantly Affecting Blood Sugar Levels. Examples Include:

- Leafy Greens (Spinach, Kale, Lettuce)
- Cruciferous Vegetables (Broccoli, Cauliflower, Brussels Sprouts)
- Zucchini
- Bell Peppers
- Asparagus
- Mushrooms

• **Limit High-Carb Vegetables:** While Non-Starchy Vegetables Are Encouraged, Be Mindful Of High-Carb Vegetables Such As Potatoes, Sweet Potatoes, And Carrots. Use Them In Moderation Or Choose Lower-Carb Alternatives.

• **Control Portion Sizes:** Pay Attention To Portion Sizes, Especially If Weight Loss Is A Goal. While Low-Carb Foods Can Be Filling, It's Still Essential To Consume An Appropriate Amount Of Calories For Your Needs.

• **Incorporate Herbs And Spices:** Enhance The Flavor Of Your Meals With Herbs And Spices, As They Add Taste Without Contributing Significant Carbs Or Calories. Examples Include

Basil, Oregano, Cumin, Garlic, And Turmeric.

- **Include Low-Carb Snacks:** Choose Snacks That Align With A Low-Carb Lifestyle, Such As Cheese, Nuts, Seeds, Or Vegetables With Dip. Be Mindful Of Portion Sizes To Avoid Overeating.

- **Stay Hydrated:** Drink Plenty Of Water Throughout The Day. Sometimes, Thirst Can Be Mistaken For Hunger, And Staying Hydrated Is Essential For Overall Health.

Here Is An Example Of A Well-Balanced Low-Carbohydrate Meal:

Grilled Chicken Breast (Protein)

- Broccoli Cooked In Olive Oil (Non-Starchy Veggie)

• Quinoa Or Cauliflower Rice (Optional, Based On Carbohydrate Tolerance)

• Mixed Greens Side Salad with Cherry Tomatoes and Avocado (Rich In Healthy Fats)

Keep In Mind That Each Person's Carbohydrate Tolerance Differs, So You May Have To Modify Portion Sizes And Meal Selections According To Your Preferences And Health Objectives. For Specialized Advise About Specific Health Concerns Or Dietary Needs, It Is Advisable To Consult With A Healthcare Expert Or A Qualified Dietitian.

Choosing the Right Foods

To Follow A Low-Carb Lifestyle, Focus On Nutrient-Dense Natural Foods And Limit Processed And High-Carb Options. Here Are Some Tips To Assist You In Making Well-Informed Decisions:

Protein Sources:

Choose Lean Protein Sources Such As:

- Poultry (Chicken, Turkey)
- Lean Cuts Of Beef, Pork, Or Lamb
- Fish And Seafood
- Eggs
- Tofu Or Tempeh (For Vegetarians)

- Dairy Products (Greek Yogurt, Cottage Cheese, Cheese)

Healthy Fats:

Include Sources Of Healthy Fats, Such As:

- Avocado Or Guacamole
- Olive Oil
- Coconut Oil
- Nuts And Seeds (Almonds, Walnuts, Chia Seeds)
- Fatty Fish (Salmon, Mackerel, Sardines)
- Butter Or Ghee (In Moderation)

Non-Starchy Vegetables:

Prioritize Non-Starchy Vegetables, Which Are Low In Carbs And High In

Fiber And Nutrients. Examples Include:

- Leafy Greens (Spinach, Kale, Lettuce)
- Cruciferous Vegetables (Broccoli, Cauliflower, Brussels Sprouts)
- Zucchini
- Bell Peppers
- Asparagus
- Mushrooms

Low-Sugar Fruits:

If You Choose To Include Fruits, Opt For Those With Lower Sugar Content, Such As:

- Berries (Strawberries, Blueberries, Raspberries)

- Avocado
- Lemon Or Lime

Whole Grains (In Moderation Or Low-Carb Alternatives):

If You Include Grains, Choose Whole Grains Or Lower-Carb Alternatives Like:

- Quinoa
- Cauliflower Rice
- Zucchini Noodles (Zoodles)
- Almond Or Coconut Flour (For Baking)

Dairy:

Choose Full-Fat Or Low-Fat Dairy Products, Such As:

- Greek Yogurt (Unsweetened)

- Cheese

- Heavy Cream (In Moderation)

Herbs and Spices: Use Herbs And Spices To Add Flavor Without Added Carbs Or Calories. Examples Include Basil, Oregano, Cumin, Garlic, And Turmeric.

Sugar Substitutes (If Desired): If You Have A Sweet Tooth, Consider Using Sugar Substitutes Like Stevia, Erythritol, Or Monk Fruit In Moderation.

Snacks: Opt For Low-Carb Snacks Such As:

- Cheese Sticks Or Slices
- Nuts And Seeds

- Vegetables With Dip (Guacamole, Hummus)

Read Labels: Be Vigilant About Reading Food Labels To Identify Hidden Sugars, High-Carb Additives, And Processed Ingredients.

It Is Important To Keep In Mind That Each Person's Tolerance To Carbohydrates Is Different. Therefore, It Is Crucial To Select Foods That Support Your Particular Health Objectives And Choices. If You Have Particular Health Issues Or Dietary Requirements, It Is Advisable To Get Advice And Direction From A Healthcare Practitioner Or A Licensed Dietitian.

CHAPTER FOUR
Dining Out On a Low-Carb Diet

Enjoying A Good Dinner While Adhering To A Low-Carb Diet Can Be Achieved Via Careful Planning And Making Wise Decisions When Dining Out. Here Are Some Guidelines For Browsing Restaurant Menus When Following A Low-Carb Diet:

• **Choose Protein-Based Options:** Look For Dishes That Feature Protein-Rich Foods Such As Grilled Chicken, Fish, Steak, Or Other Lean Meats. These Choices Can Help You Stay Full And Satisfied Without Consuming Excess Carbs.

• **Opt For Grilled Or Roasted Preparations:** Choose Grilled, Roasted, Or Baked Dishes Instead Of Fried Options. These Cooking Methods Typically Involve Fewer Added Carbs And Fats.

• **Skip The Bread Basket Or Ask For Alternatives:** Avoid Bread, Rolls, Or Tortilla Chips That Are Often Served As Appetizers. If You Enjoy A Starter, Consider Options Like A Salad Or A Vegetable-Based Appetizer.

• **Replace Starchy Sides:** Request Substitutions For High-Carb Side Dishes. For Example, Swap Out Potatoes Or Rice For Extra Vegetables Or A Side Salad. Many Restaurants Are

Willing To Accommodate Such Requests.

• **Order Salads with Protein:** Salads Can Be A Great Low-Carb Option, But Be Cautious With Dressings And Toppings. Choose Salads With A Variety Of Vegetables, Add Protein (Grilled Chicken, Shrimp, Or Steak), And Opt For A Dressing On The Side To Control The Amount You Use.

• **Check For Hidden Carbs In Sauces:** Be Mindful Of Sauces And Dressings, As They Can Often Contain Hidden Sugars And Carbs. Ask For Sauces On The Side Or Inquire About Low-Carb Options.

- **Asian Cuisine Tips:** When Dining At Asian Restaurants, Choose Stir-Fries With Lean Protein And Lots Of Vegetables. Ask For No Rice Or Noodles, Or Request A Substitution With Cauliflower Rice.

- **Mexican Cuisine Tips:** For Mexican Cuisine, Opt For Fajitas Without The Tortillas, Or Order A Salad With Grilled Meat, Cheese, Guacamole, And Salsa.

- **Italian Cuisine Tips:** Italian Restaurants Can Be Tricky, But You Can Choose Protein-Rich Dishes Like Grilled Fish Or Chicken. Skip Pasta And Ask For A Vegetable Side Instead.

- **Drink Water Or Unsweetened Tea:** Opt For Water, Unsweetened Tea, Or Black Coffee Instead Of Sugary Beverages. This Helps Avoid Unnecessary Carb Intake.

- **Review The Menu Online:** Check The Restaurant's Menu Online Before You Go. This Allows You To Plan Your Order In Advance And Avoid Impulsive High-Carb Choices.

- **Communicate Dietary Preferences:** Don't Hesitate To Communicate Your Dietary Preferences And Restrictions To The Server. Most Restaurants Are Willing To Accommodate Special Requests.

Flexibility Is Important, And It's Acceptable To Occasionally Modify Based On Your Preferences And Social Circumstances. It Is Possible To Dine Out And Adhere To A Low-Carb Lifestyle By Making Thoughtful Decisions And Planning Ahead.

Physical Activity with a Diet Low in Carbohydrates

Physical Activity Can Enhance A Low-Carbohydrate Lifestyle And Promote General Health And Wellness. Here Are Some Factors To Consider When Adding Exercise To A Low-Carb Lifestyle:

1. Energy Source: - On A Low-Carb Diet, the Body Predominantly Utilizes Fats for Energy. Regular Physical

Activity Enhances Fat Usage For Energy, Which Complements The Concepts Of Low-Carb Lifestyle.

2. Aerobic Workouts Including Walking, Jogging, Cycling, And Swimming Can Be Advantageous For Individuals Following A Low-Carb Diet. These Activities Improve Cardiovascular Health, Aid In Burning Calories, And Can Assist In Weight Control.

3. Strength Training: Including Strength Training In Your Regimen Is Crucial For Developing And Preserving Lean Muscle Mass. Preserving Muscle Mass Can Be Particularly Advantageous When Adhering To A

Low-Carb Diet For Weight Loss, As It Helps Increase Metabolic Rate.

4. High-Intensity Interval Training (HIIT) Consists Of Brief Periods Of Intensive Exercise Alternated With Short Rest Intervals. This Workout Modality Is Efficient For Calorie Expenditure, Boosting Cardiovascular Health, And Improving Insulin Sensitivity.

5. Incorporating Exercises That Emphasize Flexibility And Mobility, Like Yoga Or Pilates, Can Enhance Joint Health, Lower The Likelihood Of Injuries, And Boost General Well-Being.

6. Post-Exercise Nutrition: After Exercising, It Is Crucial To Address Your Nutritional Requirements. Following A Low-Carb Diet Requires Replenishing Electrolytes And Consuming Sufficient Protein For Muscle Regeneration.

7. Hydration Is Essential, Particularly While Adhering To A Low-Carbohydrate Diet. Water Is Crucial For Maintaining Good Health And Can Enhance Physical Performance.

8. Individualized Approach: The Most Suitable Style And Level Of Exercise May Differ From Person To Person. Take Into Account Your Fitness Level, Preferences, And Any

Preexisting Health Concerns While Selecting Your Exercise Regimen.

9. Monitoring Blood Glucose Levels: If You Have Diabetes Or Are Regulating Blood Sugar Levels, Track Your Blood Glucose Levels Before And After Exercise To Comprehend Your Body's Reactions. Modifications To Medications Or Carbohydrate Consumption May Be Required.

10. Consistency Is Key For Long-Term Health Advantages When It Comes To Establishing A Regular Workout Regimen. Discover Enjoyable Activities To Integrate Fitness As A Lasting Component Of Your Routine.

Prior To Commencing A New Workout Routine, Particularly If You Have Current Health Issues, It Is Recommended To Get Guidance From A Healthcare Provider Or A Fitness Specialist. They May Offer Personalized Instruction And Ensure That Your Workout Regimen Is In Line With Your Low-Carb Lifestyle Objectives.

Ensuring Sustained Success over an Extended Period

To Sustain Long-Term Success With A Low-Carb Lifestyle, It Is Important To Develop Enduring Behaviors That Promote General Health And Well-Being. Here Are Some Crucial Strategies To Help You Achieve And Maintain Success In The Long Run:

1. Emphasize Consuming Full, Nutrient-Dense Foods That Offer Important Nutrients, Avoiding Processed Options. Incorporate A Diverse Selection Of Vegetables, Lean Meats, Healthy Fats, And, If Manageable, Small Servings Of Whole Grains Or Legumes.

2. Maintain A Balanced Diet Of Macronutrients, Such As Proteins, Lipids, And Carbohydrates. Although Carbohydrates Are Limited, It Is Crucial To Ensure Sufficient Intake Of Fiber And Minerals For Overall Well-Being.

3. Practice Portion Control By Being Mindful Of Serving Sizes To Prevent Overeating, Even While Consuming Low-Carb Foods. Utilize Visual Indicators, Like A Well-Proportioned Plate With Protein, Veggies, And Fats, To Determine Appropriate Portion Proportions.

4. Maintain Proper Hydration By Consuming A Sufficient Quantity Of Water During The Day. Feelings Of

Hunger Can Occasionally Be Confused With Dehydration. Ensuring Proper Hydration Is Crucial For Maintaining Good Health And Can Aid In Managing Weight.

5. Engage In Consistent Physical Activity That Suits Your Fitness Level And Preferences. Engaging In Cardiovascular Workouts, Weight Training, And Flexibility Exercises Collectively Enhances One's General Well-Being.

6. Incorporate Social Support By Sharing Your Goals With Friends Or Family Members Who Can Offer Encouragement And Support. Building A Community Of Individuals With

Similar Health Objectives Can Be Inspiring And Beneficial.

7. Plan And Prepare Meals By Organizing And Cooking Them At Home Whenever Feasible. This Enables You To Have Improved Management Of The Ingredients And Portion Amounts.

8. Engage In Mindful Eating By Paying Attention To Your Hunger And Fullness Signals. Consume Your Meal At A Leisurely Pace, Relishing The Flavors And Textures While Being Mindful Of Each Bite.

9. Monitor And Adapt Your Approach Regularly Based On Your Body's Response And Health Goals.

10. Employ A Flexible And Responsive Approach. Life Events And Circumstances May Occur That Test Your Nutritional Decisions. Learn To Adapt Without Remorse And Concentrate On Making Healthier Decisions In The Future.

11. Acknowledge And Appreciate Accomplishments That Go Beyond Weight Measurements, Such As More Energy, Improved Mood, Better Sleep, And Overall Enhanced Well-Being.

12. Seek Help From Healthcare Specialists Or Licensed Dietitians If Necessary. They Offer Customized Guidance And Assistance In Resolving Any Particular Issues Or Obstacles You Encounter.

Long-Term Success Hinges On Establishing A Sustainable And Fulfilling Lifestyle. It's Important To Establish Behaviors That Enhance Your General Well-Being And Joy, Rather Than Just Adhering To A Diet. Pay Attention To Your Body, Practice Patience, And Prioritize Decisions That Promote Your Long-Term Well-Being.

Conclusion

Ultimately, Transitioning To A Low-Carb Lifestyle Requires Making Deliberate Decisions Regarding The Quality And Quantity Of Carbohydrates Taken, With A Focus On Nutrient-Rich Meals. Low-Carb Diets Can Be Advantageous For Weight Loss, Blood Sugar Management, And Overall Health When Practiced With Equilibrium And Long-Term Viability.

• Important Factors To Consider Are Including Lean Proteins, Healthy Fats, And Non-Starchy Veggies In Meals, While Being Aware Of Portion Proportions. Emphasizing Whole, Unprocessed Foods Helps Create A Balanced And Nutritious Diet. Physical

Activity Is Essential For Enhancing A Low-Carb Diet, Promoting General Health, And Assisting With Weight Control.

• Long-Term Success Requires Developing Lasting Habits, Staying Hydrated, Exercising Regularly, And Obtaining Social Support When Necessary. Tracking Advancements, Acknowledging Achievements Beyond Weight, And Being Flexible In Response To Life's Fluctuations All Enhance A Beneficial And Enduring Low-Carbohydrate Lifestyle.

Individual Responses To Dietary Modifications Can Vary, Therefore It's Recommended To Get Tailored Assistance From Healthcare

Specialists Or Registered Dietitians, Especially If You Have Specific Health Issues Or Medical Conditions.

A Low-Carb Lifestyle Focuses On Building A Balanced And Pleasurable Way Of Eating That Aligns With Your Health Goals And Increases Your General Well-Being, Rather Than Just Restricting Certain Foods.

THE END